WILD YAM:
Nature's Progesterone

THE SAFE ANSWER TO HORMONAL IMBALANCE, PMS,
MENOPAUSE AND OSTEOPOROSIS

by Rita Elkins, M.A.

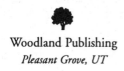

Woodland Publishing
Pleasant Grove, UT

Note: This brief and easy to understand booklet explores the uses of natural progesterone for a myriad of symptoms women continually endure assuming that their only option is synthetic hormone therapy. Issues pertaining to menstrual disorders, PMS, fibrocystic breasts, menopausal miseries, osteoporosis, and cancer are discussed supporting the use of safe, natural forms of progesterone from plant precursors. Natural progesterone may be the most valuable supplement a woman can take during the course of her life.

The information in this book is for educational purposes only and is not recommended as a means of diagnosing or treating an illness. All matters concerning physical and mental health should be supervised by a health practitioner knowledgeable in treating that particular illness. Neither the publisher nor author directly or indirectly dispense medical advice, nor do they prescribe any remedies or assume any responsibility for those who choose to treat themselves.

Contents

Progesterone: Ignorance Is Not Bliss

Has anyone ever asked you if you might be suffering from a progesterone deficiency? Women ranging in age from 12 to 100 may be subject to low progesterone levels and as a result, can suffer from a whole host of mysterious ills related to a hormonal imbalance. While most women are fairly informed about birth control pills and estrogen replacement therapy with all of its controversy, few of us understand the very profound role progesterone plays in determining our overall health. Moreover, the therapeutic effects of natural progesterone remain relatively unknown and untapped.

Of even more significance is that a growing number of women seem to be suffering from progesterone depletion and estrogen dominance. If you're like I was, this notion struck me as a completely new concept. I can say now, in retrospect, that this bit of knowledge is clearly one of the most important pieces of information I have had the opportunity to research.

So many symptoms that women have to endure are readily branded as just part of inevitable PMS or worse yet, products of an overactive imagination or emerging psychosis. It is has been through my own personal experience with terrible mood swings, horrendous periods and all sorts of miserable hormonal demons that I have come to write this booklet. Make no mistake however, the information contained herein is based on scientific fact and is backed by the experience of medical doctors. More than any other physician or scientist, Dr. John R. Lee, M.D. has pioneered and documented his remarkable results using natural progesterone from wild yam for his female patients. To say the very least, his findings have profound health implications for all women.

Natural plant-based progesterone may well be the most important breakthrough therapy for women to come out of the latter twentieth century. Ironically, its use from botanical sources has a long tried and true history. Like so many valuable natural treatments, the value of plant-based progesterones have been virtually ignored by modern medical practices.

Unfortunately, most physicians focus on the use of synthetic estrogen or artificial progestins to manage female disorders such as osteoporosis when, in reality, progesterone may be the key hormone. Ironically, natural progesterone, unlike its pharmaceutical counterparts, offers an impressive array of therapeutic actions with complete safety and efficacy.

As previously mentioned, mainstream medicine continues to overlook the use of natural phytoestrogens which can offer practical treatment of hormonally-related disorders without negative side effects. These simple plant-based medicinals have been used for generations by women of almost every culture and for good reason. These botanicals have been able to support the special health needs of both pre-and post-menopausal women with little or no side effects.

Progesterone plays a profoundly more critical role in the maintenance of female health than previously assumed. Too little of this vital female hormone can lead to all kinds of menstrual disorders, infertility, miscarriages, osteoporosis and even cancer. Progesterone deficiencies are much more common that most of us would assume, even in younger women.

Replenishing progesterone in its natural form is a safe and effective way of relieving a whole host of female symptoms ranging from the mildly annoying to the seriously debilitating. Simply stated: there are viable alternatives to popping synthetic hormones for problems like PMS or menopausal distress. In many cases, specific plant-based hormone creams can achieve better results without the significant health risks associated with synthetic hormonal analogues.

Today, the use of natural progesterone is dramatically growing as women and health practitioners alike become disillusioned with synthetic hormonal therapies. Using pharmaceutical estrogen has proven to be rather disappointing in treating osteoporosis.[1] In addition, the controversy over the safety of birth control pills and estrogen replacement therapy for post-menopause rages on. In the midst of much misinformation concerning artificial hormonal drugs, plants like wild yam are being reconsidered and reevaluated for their intrinsic value.

Ironically, modern technological manipulations of these natural phytochemicals has resulted in more potency and more risk to the human body which was not designed to cope with artificial compounds. It turns out that ancient civilizations who turned to botanicals for female ills understood the value of natural therapies. In the face of high-tech pharmaceutical imitations, it turns out that Mother Nature knew what she was doing after all.

THE PRECARIOUS ACT OF BALANCING HORMONES

The very delicate relationship between progesterone and estrogen levels is what creates hormonal balance. Today we frequently hear the phrase, "she's suffering from a hormonal imbalance." What exactly does a hormonal imbalance imply, and why is it so prevalent among women of all ages? The simple truth is that our twentieth-century life style creates a great deal of health risks not previously experienced by earlier generations. Many of these new, modern factors adversely effect our endocrine systems, not to mention our overall health as well. Consequently, when we need to synthesize certain levels of progesterone, we may be lacking the proper nutrients or, as may be the case with women who have used birth control pills, our ovarian functions may be impaired. As a result, an excess of estrogen may develop predisposing us to a number of unpleasant symptoms.

Unprecedented degrees of mental stress combined with exposure to toxins, pollutants, preservatives, chemicals, and drugs can impair a woman's ability to produce progesterone. In addition, the consumption of sugary foods lacking in whole grains, overcooked, over processed, and fatty foods devoid of the raw enzymes we were meant to ingest can also wreak havoc with our glandular health. The consumption of hormonally fattened beef and poultry is certainly a concern, and may explain why premature puberty occurs in some children who are exposed to unnatural sources of animal estrogen.

Why is there more infertility now that ever before? Why do seemingly healthy young women suffer from all sorts of menstrual disorders and unprecedented levels of PMS? Why is osteoporosis such a threat today, and why is breast cancer killing so many relatively young women? Why do so many of us plow through perimenopause and postmenopause, perplexed by a wide variety of ills that threaten our emotional and physical well-being?

All of these questions are profoundly linked to hormonal factors and almost always reflect an estrogen dominance and a progesterone deficiency. I did not know that such a scenario even existed and like most women, did not understand that too much of certain kinds of estrogen can be extremely harmful. Furthermore, because I assumed that estrogen levels continued to decline as I got older, I never considered the possibility of a pre-menopausal estrogen overload. It is crucial to remember that when estrogen is unopposed by adequate levels of progesterone, a hormonal imbalance occurs. Unopposed estrogen is undesirable to say the least, and explains why so many women suffer from estrogen-related ills even as they approach menopause.

Estrogen: The Hidden Culprit

As mentioned, many women who suffer from a whole myriad of perplexing and distressing symptoms can be unsuspecting victims of an estrogen dominance. It is important to keep in mind that when estrogen is not balanced out by adequate amounts of progesterone, a whole array of diverse symptoms may develop, many of which are easily misdiagnosed and subsequently, mistreated.

In addition, we hear so much about keeping our estrogen levels up as we approach menopause, we rarely consider the fact that we may be suffering from an estrogen overload during pre-menopausal years. Most physicians neglect to discuss the very real effect of an estrogen dominance, but I can assure you that it is all too real. Enduring very heavy periods, developing sore and tender breasts, retaining water, bloating and serious bouts with depression are more of a problem for many pre-menopausal women in their forties than one would assume.

In addition, most of us are unaware of the fact that a woman can have regular periods and not be ovulating. A continued lack of ovulation or impaired ovulation can also create a progesterone deficiency leading to an abnormal buildup of the uterine lining which is never sufficiently shed. The incomplete removal of the endometrium can lead to endometriosis, uterine fibroid cysts, fibrocystic breasts, bloating, depression, heavy or irregular periods and possible malignancies.

IS ALL ESTROGEN BAD?

Certainly, all estrogen is not bad; however, it would seem that most women suffer from a dominance of estrogen and a lack of progesterone. Estrogen is the hormone that initiates female puberty, causing the development of the breast, uterus, fallopian tubes etc. It also contributes to female fat distribution. Prior to menopause, estrogen levels drop causing an eventual cessation of the menstrual period.

Most conventional physicians will recommend estrogen replacement therapy to offset the risk of osteoporosis and to prevent cardiovascular disease, two actions which are still questioned in many scientific circles. The focus on estrogen therapy may be misguided in many cases. More and more evidence points to the fact that when progesterone levels are where they should be, conditions like PMS, osteoporosis, etc. dramatically improve. Unopposed or synthetic estrogen poses a number of health risks which most women will recognize immediately through their own personal experience.

THE NEGATIVE EFFECTS OF ESTROGEN

While estrogen balanced with progesterone is necessary for proper female development and reproduction, when is dominates, it can contribute to a number of unwanted reactions, including:

- *increases body fat stores, especially on upper thighs*
- *promotes water and sodium retention in the cells*
- *contribute to impaired blood sugar levels*
- *increase the risk of endometrial (uterine) and breast cancer*
- *increase blood clotting which raises the risk of stroke*
- *contribute to mood swings*
- *thickens the bile increasing the risk of gallbladder disease*
- *cause headaches*
- *promotes the loss of zinc*
- *interferes with thyroid function*
- *contribute to excess and irregular menstrual bleeding*
- *decrease libido*
- *reduce cellular oxygenation*

SYMPTOMS OF AN ESTROGEN DOMINANCE

Aside from having your blood or saliva tested, it is relatively easy to assess whether or not you may be suffering from an estrogen dominance. The following symptoms are typical of excess estrogen and progesterone depletion: breast enlargement and tenderness, water retention, heavy menstrual flow or irregular periods, carbohydrate cravings, weight gain (fat on hips and thighs), fibrocystic breasts, uterine fibroids, loss of libido, PMS, mood swings/depression, and certain types of acne.

The Role of Naturally Occurring Progesterone in the Body

In light of the previous section, it is vital to keep in mind that when progesterone is produced and maintained, most of the negative side effects of estrogen are neutralized. Unfortunately, in far too many women, progesterone levels fail to do the job. Let's discuss exactly what progesterone is responsible for.

A woman's ovaries produce two key hormones: estrogen and progesterone during her ovulatory years. The corpus luteum makes progesterone just before ovulation which rapidly escalates during the two week period following ovulation. The primary task of progesterone is to support implantation and sustain pregnancy. It does this by inhibiting uterine contraction and by suppressing the immune system's response to the developing embryo as a foreign body.[2]

During the last two weeks of a woman's menstrual cycle, progesterone is considered the dominant female hormone. During pregnancy, the placenta takes over the task of progesterone synthesis. Progesterone is also made in limited amounts in the adrenal glands of both men and women and in the testes of the male.

PROGESTERONE SECRETION RATES

The following breakdown gives general guidelines of amounts and time of progesterone secretion:

- just before ovulation.............2 to 3 mg per day
- just after ovulation.............20 to 25 mg per day
- one week post ovulation.............30 mg per day
- during the 3rd trimester of pregnancy.....300-400 mg per day

Women who feel physically exhilarated and sometimes experience an unusual remission of diseases like bronchial asthma during pregnancy may be responding to elevated progesterone levels which help to boost the production of natural cortisone.

Approximately twelve days following ovulation, if fertilization has not occurred, progesterone levels decline rapidly, which initiates the shedding of the uterine lining, also known as menstruation.

In time, progesterone is transported through the bloodstream to the liver where it is metabolized and excreted as waste through the kidneys (urine) and the bile. Typically, pregnancy tests are reacting to increased levels of HCG or of progesterone in the urine, indicating that pregnancy has occurred. (*Note:* What is crucial to remember is that a woman's cycle, regardless of her age, may not be characterized by the above scale. A number of factors may cause estrogen to remain dominant, even after progesterone is supposed to take over in the latter half of the cycle. Even young women who suffer from nutritional deficiencies, stress, etc. may experience an estrogen dominance, suggesting the need for natural progesterone supplementation.)

The Three-fold Action of Progesterone

1. It ensures the implantation and development of a fertilized egg and subsequent embryo and fetus.

2. It acts as a precursor to other steroid hormones such as cortisone which is produced in the adrenal glands and contributes to the production of the sex hormones including testosterone.

3. It exerts a number of desirable physiological actions.

Botanical Progesterone: What Is It?

Simply stated, certain plants exist in nature which contain both estrogens and progesterone very similar to those produced in the human body. These botanicals are referred to as "phytoestrogens" and number in the thousands. Some of these plants include soybeans and mistletoe, however, one of the most abundant sources of progesterone is contained in diosgenin which is found in wild yam (dioscorea). Wild yam provides the source of a cost effective and safe form of progesterone. Natural progesterone is primarily produced from wild yam.

By contrast, synthetic progesterone preparations should technically be referred to as progestogens. Both Premarin and Provera are commonly prescribed for hormonal imbalances, after a hysterectomy or during menopause. Premarin is actually an altered form of estrogen (conjugated) and Provera is not technically a progesterone but a synthetic analogue (progestin).

WILD YAM: NATURE'S ANSWER TO HORMONAL IMBALANCES

In 1985 Rudolf Weiss wrote, "Wild yams contain diosgenin, a precursor in the synthesis of progesterone, and are the only known available source."[3] Mexican wild yam is the richest phytoestrogen available and provides the human body with a natural and safe source of progesterone. It has an anti-spasmodic action which make is ideal for treating menstrual cramping and is an excellent contributor to achieving glandular balance. Native Americans have used wild yam for generations for the treatment of female disorders and as a supportive herbal for pregnancy.

In 1936, Japanese scientists discovered the glycoside saponins found in several wild yam species from which steroid saponins (diosgenin) could be extracted.[4] Diosgenin is remarkably similar to progesterone it its chemical configuration. Because of its steroidal saponins, wild yam has been used for hundreds of prescription drugs including some birth control pills; however, these forms of the plant have been chemically isolated and altered resulting in variations of the plant's natural compounds. These artificially manipulated chemicals can initiate abnormal responses in the human body, a fact which accounts for their long list of risks and side effects. Synthetic forms of progesterone whether derived from wild yam or not are not the same as an extract of the whole wild yam. It's useful to know that products listing wild yam as an ingredient may not included the saponin-rich portion of the yam root.

Progesterone which is derived from wild yam is almost identical in its chemical structure to the natural progesterone synthesized by the human body. When wild yam is absorbed into the body it is easily converted into the same molecule, a process which does not occur with synthetic varieties. The transition is easy and natural.

Wild yam in and of itself does not contain simple progesterone or other steroids, but serves as a precursor to these compounds. The phytoestrogen character of wild yam explains its traditional usage for menstrual cramping, dysmenorrhea, and afterbirth pains.

NATURAL VS. PHARMACEUTICAL PROGESTERONE

Due to its marketability, pharmaceutical companies looked to patentable progesterone analogues which were chemically synthesized from the progesterone derived from the wild yam. This new class of drugs were called progestins or prestrogens and while they may have originated from the wild yam, they differed profoundly in their overall biological action as well as their toxicity. These enhanced and chemically synthesized versions of wild yam progesterone did not offer the total and synergistic effects wild yam provided in its natural state. Furthermore, they posed significant health risks which many women are not completely aware of. While synthetic progestin drugs pose health hazards, natural progesterone does not.[5]

SIDE EFFECTS OF SYNTHETIC PROGESTIN DRUGS

Premarin and Provera are two of the most commonly prescribed progestin drugs and come with a wide variety of side effects and health risks. Over 30 negative side effects are listed for Provera alone. Taking Provera during early pregnancy may actually cause a miscarriage or deformity of the developing fetus. Premarin is comprised of two different types of estrogen called estrone and estradiol, which have been linked with the development of certain kinds of cancer.

The risks involved with taking these synthetic progestins is due to their chemical structures. For the most part, the compound resembles natural progesterone, therefore it binds to the same receptor sites as to natural progesterone. The altered portions of the molecule, however, convey a totally different signal to the cells involved. It is this atomic manipulation which poses alarming health risks to the body. Health risks which are not associated with natural hormonal precursors. A few of the side effects associated with synthetic progestins include:

- *increased risk of cancer*
- *migraines*
- *breast tenderness*
- *changes in cholesterol levels*
- *blood sugar disorders*
- *high blood pressure*
- *birth defects*

- *fluid retention*
- *kidney problems*
- *blood clots*
- *menstrual irregularities*
- *weight gain*
- *depression*
- *miscarriage*

As is often the case, eventually the perils of synthetically derived plant analogues made health practitioners question their usage and the notion of using progesterone in its natural state has re-emerged. Unfortunately, its classification as a non-patentable simple substance relegates it to the status of an herbal supplement, which most doctors will not endorse. Synthetic drugs are more potent, usually easier to take, have a longer physiologic action and are patentable. For all of these reasons, natural phytomedicines have been shelved as relatively worthless in comparison. Chemically altered progesterone is considered technically superior when in reality, natural forms of progesterone may often be preferable.

OTHER BIOLOGIC BENEFITS OF NATURAL PROGESTERONE

While natural progesterone has been referred to as a progestin because it maintains the lining of the uterus, it is technically separate and totally different from synthetic progestins. In addition, natural progesterone provides a number of biological actions which progestins do not. Some additional benefits reported with the use of natural progesterone include:

- *reduction in joint pain and swelling*
- *enhanced skin moisturization*
- *fading of liver spots*
- *faster healing of wounds*
- *reduction of yeast infections*
- *supports the immune system*
- *protects against the side effects of unopposed estrogen*
- *tranquilizing*
- *sleep promotion*

THERAPEUTIC APPLICATIONS OF NATURAL PROGESTERONE

- *necessary for the survival and development of the fetus*
- *helps to prevent osteoporosis*
- *needed for the proper production of adrenal hormones*
- *works to stabilize blood sugar*
- *has a natural diuretic action*
- *prevents salt retention*
- *acts as an antidepressant*
- *helps prevent the formation of fibrocystic breasts*
- *enhances thermogenesis (the burning of fat)*
- *contributes to regulating the thyroid gland*
- *enhances libido*
- *helps protect the uterus and breasts from malignancies*
- *contributes to blood clotting mechanisms*
- *precursor of corticosterones*
- *helps to protect against breast cancer*
- *normalizes zinc and copper levels*
- *maintains the secretory endometrium*

Note: Using natural progesterone in cream, oil or other transdermal form is also very hydrating to the skin.

SAFETY OF NATURAL PROGESTERONE

Natural progesterone is one of the safest supplements available. In contrast to synthetic progestins, this form of progesterone has little or no side effects. Some women may experience an initial reaction to introducing progesterone, a phenomenon which involves an estrogen response. In these cases, estrogen-related symptoms may temporarily become worse. If this occurs, natural progesterone should be continued or dosages adjusted until hormonal balance is achieved. Incidental spotting between periods may occur but is usually resolved within three to five cycles. The use of natural progesterone has not been linked to any form of human cancer.

Combining natural progesterone with other drugs has not resulted in any interference or alteration that is known of. No adverse effects of natural progesterone have been reported on the developing fetus of pregnant women, unlike its synthetic counterparts. Using natural progesterone creams during pregnancy appears to be perfectly safe and may even help to counteract the post-partum depression which so many women experience after their progesterone levels fall dramatically. (*Note:* When natural progesterone is first introduced into the body, an initial estrogen response may occur possibly making estrogen-related symptoms more intense. This reaction is perfectly normal and varies with each individual. It is a temporary phenomenon and continued use will eventually achieve hormonal balance. Experiencing longer periods, heavier flows, more cramping, tender breasts etc. may indicate that natural progesterone dosages may need to be adjusted in order to achieve hormonal balance.)

WHY TOPICAL APPLICATION OF NATURAL PROGESTERONE?

Progesterone is a fat soluble compound which maintains its integrity much more readily when absorbed transdermally (through the skin) than when taken my mouth. When progesterone is ingested orally, it is subject to rapid breakdown (metabolism) in the liver, making it considerably less effective. Medical practitioners have used synthetic progesterone in a variety of forms

ranging from capsules to injections to vaginal and rectal supposi-
tories.

Originally, orally administered progesterone or progestins were
not efficiently absorbed through the intestinal wall and had to pass
through liver tissue before entering the bloodstream. Consequently, much of the absorbed progestins were metabolized by the
liver into inactive compounds. Up to 80 percent of the effectiveness of progesterone can be lost when taken orally.[6] By contrast,
progesterone is very nicely absorbed transdermally (through the
skin) and much more of its biochemical activity is retained.

> I believe that natural progesterone cream derived from wild yam
> extract should be used by almost every mature adult . . . I believe that
> progesterone cream could do more to preserve health and well-being
> in elderly people than all the drugs in the world.[7]

Dr. Lee reiterates that ". . . natural progesterone is efficiently
absorbed transdermally, a fact that enhances patient's acceptance of
its use and greatly reduces the cost of therapy."[8]

Salivary hormonal lab tests are becoming more common and
have further supported the effectiveness of natural progesterone
absorption through the skin by monitoring levels.[9] These tests have
proven that progesterone levels rise when wild yam extracts are
applied to the skin.

Natural Progesterone and PMS

When a woman's body experiences an imbalance of progesterone resulting in estrogen dominance, a variety of pre-menstrual
symptoms can result. Estrogen dominance can occur when a progesterone deficiency is present. PMS refers to a whole host of symptoms which can vary from woman to woman. Conventional therapies for PMS involves the use of antidepressants, diuretics, coun-
seling, nutritional regimens and synthetic hormones. Interestingly,
most symptoms which commonly characterize PMS are also typical of estrogen dominance. Due to this observation, Dr. John R.
Lee gave natural progesterone to his patients with PMS and

obtained some impressive results. "The majority (but not all) of such patients reported remarkable improvement in their symptoms-complex, including the elimination of their premenstrual water retention and weight gain."[10]

Let's quickly review the hormonal flux which characterizes the menstrual cycle. During the week following the end of the menstrual period, estrogen is the dominating hormone which initiates the buildup of the uterine lining once again. At the same time, eggs in the ovary begin to mature. Estrogen levels also contribute to the secretion of more vaginal mucous at this time making the tissue environment more conducive to sperm survival and motility.

From ten to twelve days after the beginning of the last period, estrogen levels will crest and then begin to taper just prior to ovulation and when the egg (corpus luteum) has matured enough to produce progesterone. Consequently, progesterone will dominate during the second half of the cycle. Increased levels of progesterone cause the body temperature to rise, the continued development of the uterine blood-filled lining, and the thinning of cervical secretions. All of these events occur in anticipation of the presence of a fertilized egg.

If pregnancy does not occur within 10 to 12 days after ovulation, both estrogen and progesterone levels rapidly fall, which initiates the shedding of the uterine lining (menstruation) and a new cycle begins again. If a woman becomes pregnant, progesterone levels continue to rise and the uterine lining remains intact to receive and nourish the fertilized egg. Eventually the placenta will produce much higher than normal amounts of progesterone throughout the remainder of the pregnancy.

It's rather easy to see that a woman's monthly cycle is regulated by the rise and fall of estrogen and progesterone. This perfectly natural fluctuation of hormones can wreak havoc with the health of a woman when imbalances occur. More often than not, a hormonal imbalance consists of a progesterone deficiency. Progesterone was designed by nature to inhibit many of the negative effects of estrogen. If progesterone levels do not balance out estrogen during the last two weeks of the cycle, PMS can become a problem. Dr. Lee illustrates this, saying: "A surplus of estrogen or a deficiency of progesterone during these two weeks allows for an abnormal month-long exposure to estrogen dominance, setting the stage for the symptoms of estrogen side effects."[11]

Clearly, natural progesterone may be one of the most, if not the most effective, therapies to deal with PMS miseries. Unfortunately, many women are completely unaware of its action or availability.

WHY DO SO MANY WOMEN SUFFER FROM HORMONE IMBALANCES?

The question of why so many women, young and old, suffer from a hormonal imbalance persists. Today's environment and life style are certainly significant causal factors and explain, to a great degree why even young, seemingly healthy women may experience a lack of progesterone. Dr. Peter Elliston of the Harvard Anthropology Department found through one of his studies of 18 women who all had regular menstrual cycles that seven of them did not experience a mid cycle increase in progesterone levels, suggesting that ovulation did not actually occur.[12] Dr. Lee cites this as yet another example of the widespread incidence of anovulatory cycles occurring in young women throughout this country, a fact which is undoubtedly linked to rising infertility rates in the United States.

Eating disorders, poor nutrition, widespread use of birth control pills, stress, pollution, etc., contribute to hormonally-related disorders and most certainly affect progesterone production, the ability to conceive and menopausal transitions.

CAUSES OF HORMONE IMBALANCES

- *stress*
- *environmental pollution*
- *ingested toxins*
- *nutritional deficiencies*
- *birth control pills*
- *synthetic hormones*
- *menopause*
- *xenoestrogens (substances which act like estrogen in the body such as*
- *certain pollutants)*
- *hormonal residue in animal meats*

It's relatively easy to determine if your hormones are out of balance and if you are lacking progesterone. One of the key symptoms of a progesterone deficiency is the presence of PMS. Even a young, relatively healthy woman can suffer from a lack of progesterone. In addition, we live in a world full of toxins, food additives and hormonally fattened meats. Dr. Lee believes that widespread use of the birth control pill has caused the ovaries to be compromised, possibly playing a role in the development of PMS that would normally not exist.[13]

Documented results from using natural progesterone have been impressive but remain relatively unknown by the majority of women. Progesterone therapy can help relieve the following PMS symptoms: breast engorgement, breast tenderness, irritability, headaches, depression, moodiness, fatigue, anxiety, bloating, water retention, cramps, and irregular periods.

Dr. Joel T. Hargrove of Vanderbilt University Medical Center has had some very impressive results using natural progesterone to treat his patients with PMS. He has had a 90 percent success rate using this form of progesterone.[14] Interestingly, he used oral progesterone which had to be administered in a much heavier dose to achieve the same results Dr. Lee obtained with transdermal progesterone.[15]

Natural Progesterone and Other Menstrual Disorders

PERIOD REGULATOR

Natural progesterone can contribute to restoring normal menstrual cycling in certain cases. Many young women suffer from amenorrhea, which is the absence of the menstrual period due to an excess of strenuous exercise or a hormonal imbalance. Using natural progesterone can help to achieve the proper estrogen/progesterone ratios needed to initiate normal cycling. Frequently, supplementation needs to occur over several months before normal cycling will be achieved.

In addition, women who suffer from irregular periods or prolonged periods can benefit from the action of natural progesterone. Remember, that initially, cycles may become worse rather than better, but with continued use, the prospect for normalizing the menstrual cycle is good if no other contributing factors exist.

THE FERTILITY LINK

Natural progesterone supplementation may also be beneficial for infertility. Women who suffer from repeated miscarriages or have a difficult time conceiving should be checked for a progesterone deficiency. It is advisable to check your progesterone levels before taking potent fertility drugs or synthetic hormones. Using natural progesterone is suggested as an initial therapy.

PROGESTERONE REPLACEMENT AND MOOD SWINGS

Consider the following quote concerning mood elevation and depression and progesterone replacement:

> The domino effect of the inter-relationship between amino acids, vitamins and neurotransmitters is further complicated by the presence of estrogen . . . an estrogen overload can cause a number of distressing symptoms. Estrogen is a central nervous system stimulant while progesterone has the opposite effect. Maintaining the right balance between these two hormones is a complex and delicate process. Any imbalance can trigger a change in mood. In order to have enough serotonin, you need tryptophan which is necessary for its production. To have enough tryptophan, your body must have certain amounts of vitamin B6. This chemical chain can be broken by estrogen, which can block the action of vitamin B6 and force it to be eliminated from the body . . . consequently, you feel like the world is coming to an end.[16]

Ironically, synthetic forms of progesterone which are routinely prescribed to help with PMS related depression etc. can actually inhibit the absorption of vitamin B6, thereby contributing to emotional instability and mood swings.

Clinical depression, anxiety attacks and mood swings can all respond to natural progesterone therapy. In addition to opposing estrogen, progesterone stimulates the adrenal glands which help to elevate mood and create energy. One of the most dramatic effects of using natural progesterone is in creating emotional stability. In other words, fluctuating between euphoria and depression in response to hormonal flux is greatly eased by increased progesterone. The short-tempered, anxious or nervous states so typical of PMS are also tempered by keeping estrogen levels in check.

FIBROCYSTIC BREASTS

The developments of fibrocystic breasts is directly linked to an excess of estrogen. One of the most dramatic therapeutic effects of natural progesterone is the rapid clearing of these types of breast cysts. Dr. Lee's experience with natural progesterone treatment for this disorder is nothing less than remarkable; he found that if natural progesterone was applied in cream form for two week prior to menstruation, fibrocystic breasts completely cleared within 2 to 3 months.[17]

UTERINE FIBROID TUMORS

Fibroid tumors of the uterus can develop when estrogen remains unopposed by progesterone and can also result from repeated cycles where ovulation fails to occur. Typically women will suffer from these fibroids approximately ten years prior to the onset of menopause. Dr. Lee's work with treating uterine fibroids once again reiterates the need for natural progesterone supplementation. He writes, "If sufficient natural progesterone is supplemented from day 12 to day 26 of the menstrual cycle, further growth of fibroids is usually prevented (and often the fibroids regress)."[18]

OVARIAN CYSTS

An ovarian cyst usually forms when follicles in the ovary fail to normally develop and subsequent release from the ovary is impaired in some way. As a result of this abnormality, hormonal balance is disrupted with typical estrogen surges resulting in the formation of a growing cyst either from the follicle or from the corpus luteum. Consider the following quote concerning cysts:

Natural progesterone, given from day 5 to day 26 of the menstrual month for 2-3 cycles, will almost routinely cause the cyst to disappear by suppressing normal FSH, LH and estrogen production, giving the ovary time to heal.[19]

Natural Progesterone and Menopause

During the thirties and forties of a woman's lifetime, progesterone production can decrease resulting in shorter intervals between periods. For example, when the ovaries produce progesterone for only 9 days rather than the normal 14, menstruation may occur every 24 days rather than the usual 28 days. In addition, low levels of progesterone coupled with an estrogen dominance can cause the lining of the uterus to build up leading to abnormally heavy menstrual flows or even spotting between periods.

Many women who are in perimenopause (the years just prior to the onset of menopause) experience these symptoms in combination with intensified PMS. Weight gain, bloating, headaches, irritability, depression, and anxiety are common complaints for women in their late thirties and throughout the forties. Frequently, these women had no cycle-related problems in their earlier years and suddenly become all to aware of a whole host of troubling symptoms. More often than not, a drop in progesterone and an estrogen overload are to blame.

Just because a woman no longer ovulates or has a menstrual cycle does not mean that she no longer needs to achieve a proper ratio of hormones. On the contrary, it is during these years that the right kind of hormonal supplementation needs to be implemented or menopausal symptoms and diseases like osteoporosis may develop. Today, estrogen replacement therapy (ERT) is recommended for many postmenopausal women with the assumption that it can help prevent heart disease, osteoporosis and possibly Alzheimer's disease. Unfortunately much controversy surrounds the prescription of synthetic hormones due to their potentially dangerous side effects.

Ideally, a far better solution would be to supply the body with the proper natural biochemical building blocks to prompt the production of natural hormones. This is where phytoestrogens or plant-based compounds such as dioscorea (wild yam) can play a profoundly important role in managing menopausal disorders such as osteoporosis.

PROGESTERONE AND OSTEOPOROSIS

At this writing, evidence points to the fact that natural progesterone may be even more effective in treating osteoporosis than estrogen replacement therapy. While this evidence is still in its initial stages, it is significant and must be considered. In 1981, Dr. John Lee conducted a landmark study evaluating the effectiveness of using natural progesterone for osteoporosis.[20] His study indicated that it is the cessation of progesterone production in postmenopausal women which causes the development of osteoporosis. Contrary to current trends, progesterone replacement, not estrogen, in fact may be the answer to preventing and treating osteoporosis. Dr. Lee's study has profound implications for all women.

In his practice, Dr. Lee applied a natural progesterone cream on one hundred postmenopausal women and eliminated their usual dose of oral Provera (a synthetic progestin). The majority of these women were in varying stages of osteoporosis. Each participant used the natural progesterone cream for several consecutive days each month over a period of three years. The results were dramatic, to say the least. In addition to preventing further height loss and eliminating aches and pains, the bone mineral density of the spine was preserved in 63 of the women. In other words, these women not only stopped the bone loss associated with osteoporosis but actually experienced an increase in bone mass which, in many cases was more dramatic than had been seen with other therapies. In addition, the incidence of bone fractures actually dropped to zero.

Dr Lee's study found that estrogen was not the panacea for bone density previously assumed. He discovered that the women who took estrogen in combination with the progesterone were not better off than those who took progesterone alone. What was even more impressive was discovering that osteoporosis is a reversible condition with progesterone therapy. Concerning the use of progesterone for osteoporosis, Dr. Lee writes:

. . . when my 40 year old housewives had become 60-year olds with osteoporosis and I learned of transdermal natural progesterone (being sold as a skin moisturizer), I started adding it to my therapeutic regimen for osteoporosis, at first only to those for whom estrogen was contraindicated. To my surprise, serial bone mineral density tests showed a significant rise without a hint of side effects. With this obvious success, my use of natural progesterone spread to osteoporosis patients who were not doing all that well on estrogen alone. Again, it proved successful.[21]

Apparently, women who had the lowest bone densities experienced the greatest increases, implying that age and the progression of the diseases does not affect the beneficial therapeutic action of natural progesterone. This study is profoundly significant in that it strongly suggests that women who take estrogen to prevent or treat osteoporosis may be better off using natural progesterone. As a result of Lee's findings, several physicians began to use natural progesterone cream for their pre- and post-menopausal patients.

The most striking implication of Dr. Lee's work with natural progesterone is that contrary to current medical opinion, osteoporosis may be more a manifestation of a progesterone deficiency than a lack of estrogen. In addition, the disease may be initiated long before menopause when estrogen levels are still high.[22] Moreover, continued estrogen therapy for women with osteoporosis often caps out whereas progesterone therapy continually promotes the production of new bone.[23] Dr. C. Norman Shealy, M.D. states:

I believe that natural progesterone cream derived from wild yam extract should be used by almost every mature adult . . . The most common cause of death in elderly women is from the complications of fracture of the hip from osteoporosis. Such fractures are also remarkably common in men. I believe that progesterone cream could do more to preserve health and well-being in elderly people than all the drugs in the world.[24]

More Benefits of Natural Progesterone

PROGESTERONE AND CANCER

The two types of cancer that are hormonally related include breast and uterine cancer due to the fact that the tissue which make up these areas are much more sensitive to hormone levels. It is a well known fact that an excess of estrogen can increase the risk of developing uterine cancer and certain types of estrogen have been linked to the formation of malignant breast tumors.[25]

Any woman who continually suffers from insufficient progesterone can also increase her chances of developing certain types of cancer. A prolonged lack of progesterone can cause uterine changes which eventually result in the impaired shedding of the uterine lining. When this occurs month after month, endometrial hyperplasia can result, which is the abnormal thickening of the uterine lining. This buildup can lead to the development of uterine cancer. Progesterone can actually reduce the risk of developing uterine cancer which can develop from using estrogen therapy.[26]

In addition, for women who have survived uterine cancer and have undergone hysterectomies, natural progesterone can be invaluable. Because these women are advised to forgo hormonal treatments of any kind, they often suffer with osteoporosis or other symptoms typical of menopause. Taking natural progesterone poses no health risks and can help to prevent or treat these disorders. Concerning this group of women Dr. Lee writes:

> These are the women for whom I first began using natural progesterone therapy. Not only did progesterone reverse their osteoporosis and, in many, it corrected their vaginal atrophy, but none, to my knowledge, have ever developed cancer of any sort . . . The evidence is overwhelming that natural progesterone is safe and only estradiol, estrone and the various synthetic estrogens and progestins are to be avoided to reduce the risk of endometrial cancer.[27]

In the case of breast cancer, studies strongly suggest that this type of malignancy is more likely to occur in premenopausal women who have normal or high estrogen levels and low progesterone levels.[28] Women over 35 who continue to have periods but no longer ovulate and women who are taking synthetic estrogen without progesterone during and after menopause may find themselves in this higher risk group.

One of the most interesting studies on progesterone was conducted at Johns Hopkins University in 1981, where physicians studied 1083 women for between 13 to 33 years in assessing the incidence of breast cancer. They found that those women who had a progesterone deficiency were over 5 times more at risk of developing breast cancer than those women who had adequate progesterone levels.[29] Moreover, the study found that women who suffered from a lack of progesterone also had ten times more cancer-related death from all types of malignancies than those who did not.[30] These statistics are dramatic, to say the least. Consider the following quote:

> . . . the evidence is strong that unopposed estradiol and estrone [two forms of estrogen] are carcinogenic for the breasts, and both progesterone and estriol, the two major hormones throughout pregnancy, are protective against breast cancer. One is left to wonder why supplementation with these two beneficial and safe hormones are not the ones used routinely for women whenever hormone supplementation seems indicated . . . both hormones are available and are relatively inexpensive. Why have these two hormones been neglected by contemporary medical practice in favor of synthetic substitutes.[31]

THE CONNECTION OF PROGESTERONE TO WEIGHT LOSS

Interestingly estrogen promotes the storing of fat and is responsible for the female contouring of the body, whereas progesterone enhances thermogenesis or fat burning. In addition, using natural progesterone to balance out hormones can help to decrease carbohydrate cravings which are hormonally related. The hormonal flux typical of most female cycles usually produces a premenstrual craving for sweets which is linked to fluctuating blood sugar and serotonin levels in the brain. Many women have found that taking natural progesterone has resulted in a marked decrease of "hormonal eating" which can result in unwanted weight gain. The desire to continually eat during periods of hormonal flux month after month certainly plays a significant role in female obesity. Excessive hormonal appetite stimulation is not normal, neither is it healthy.

Of additional interest is the fact that the more fat stores a woman carries, the more estrogen she makes, further compounding the problem. Fat cells contribute to estrogen dominance which in turn makes it harder to burn fat—a perfectly vicious little cycle. The estrogen factor for any overweight woman must be considered, however, it is rarely addressed. Clearing excess estrogen from the body is absolutely essential for effective weight loss. Again, supplementing the body with natural progesterone can help to accomplish this.

Help for Fibromyalgia?

While scientific documentation on the link between natural progesterone therapy and fibromyalgia has yet to be researched, a significant number of women are finding that the pain associated with this disorder is alleviated when taking transdermal progesterone. The cause of fibromyalgia remains a mystery to medical doctors, although its connection to hormonal factors or neurochemistry has been proposed. Taking natural progesterone has resulted in alleviating insomnia in some women, which may also be beneficial for those with fibromyalgia. The pain of fibromyalgia is especially troublesome at night.

What About Progesterone and Men?

When is comes to the role of progesterone in males, a significant inequity exists. In other words, medical science has literally ignored the role of progesterone in the male menopause. Male menopause is also called "andropause" and occurs when testosterone levels decrease. As a result of this drop, bone weakness and prostate disorders can occur.

Testosterone acts very much like progesterone explaining why men can also develop brittle bones as testosterone levels decline. Men have progesterone levels much the same as women do after the age of 50, and like women, men are subject to varying degrees of osteoporosis, although male versions are much less severe.

Men could very well benefit from using progesterone creams that have formulas designed to address testosterone imbalances which can lead to prostate disease. These formulas should contain the proper dosage of progesterone, which would be much less than the amount required for a woman. Dr. C. Norman Shealy M.D. writes, "Every male with DHEA levels below 600 ng/dl should use natural progesterone cream, except men with prostate cancer."[32] DHEA is the building block of the sex hormones and is currently the subject of intense study due to its effect on aging and degenerative disease.

How to Utilize Natural Progesterone

Natural progesterone is available in oils, capsule or cream form. The best delivery system for natural progesterone appears to be through the skin; therefore, creams, oils or other formulations designed for skin absorption are recommended. The source of the natural progesterone should be wild yam extract and preparations using the whole wild yam are preferable. Monthly costs for natural progesterone can vary according to its source, but usually average between $20 and $50 a month.

To obtain maximum absorption, natural progesterone creams should be applied to the softer areas of the skin such as the neck, face, arm pits, thighs, breasts, etc. The soles of the feet or palms of the hands are also excellent absorption sites and are recommended in individuals who are highly allergic to topical creams or oils.

A thin application over a larger area is recommended. Some women use the cream directly on their abdomens if they are experiencing menstrual cramping. Natural progesterone creams that have been combined with herbs such as saw palmetto can also be used by men and applied directly on the testicles.

Natural progesterone creams can be used every day, however, initial applications should be liberal (one half teaspoon) used both at morning and night. In time this quantity can be decreased. Using the cream everyday can lead to a decrease in sensitivity which may inhibit the action of the cream. For this reason, Dr. Lee has recommended that postmenopausal women use the cream for 2 to 3 week intervals with one week off. Women who are pre-menopausal or perimenopausal should use the progesterone from day 12 to day 26 of their menstrual cycle.

Application sites should be rotated for maximum efficacy. Leaving 3 to 5 days of the month without using the natural progesterone is also recommended to prevent the development of a kind of "immunity" to the wild yam phytoestrogens. Each individual should determine whether the amount of cream used is effective and adjust accordingly. Most women need to use natural progesterone for an indefinite period of time.

Conclusion

Natural progesterone in cream or other transdermal forms appears to be one of the most effective and safe supplements for the treatment of various hormonally related disorders. It may well be superior to estrogen replacement therapy in some cases and should be utilized and evaluated for its superior therapeutic actions. No longer the "forgotten hormone," natural progesterone, especially in the form of wild yam extract, is nothing less than remarkable in its physiological actions. While so many women are turning to synthetic hormones, tranquilizers, and analgesics to manage PMS and postmenopausal miseries, natural progesterone may well be the best and safest alternative.

Getting the word out while scientific studies continue to support the credibility of using natural progesterone is currently underway. It would be nothing less than tragic if an affordable and safe substance like wild yam extract remained unused due to a lack of knowledge. The word is spreading rapidly. Dr. Lee put it well when he stated:

> I must conclude with a tribute to what I call the women's underground communication network, the vast informal woman-to-woman communication network that spreads hormone and health information with astonishing speed and extent around the world. An informational and health revolution is underway, thanks to the networking of intelligent, concerned women.[33]

I consider myself most fortunate to have become acquainted

with natural progesterone synthesized from wild yam. For me, the discovery of this safe and marvelous supplement has been nothing less than extraordinary. It has made what was once a life lived at the mercy of the hormonal upheavals into one that is much more even-keeled, healthier and full of optimism.

Endnotes

1 John R. Lee, M.D., NATURAL PROGESTERONE: THE MULTIPLE ROLES OF A REMARK-ABLE HORMONE, Revised. (BLL Publishing, Sebastopol, California: 1993), 4. See also U.S. Barzel, "Estrogens in the prevention and treatment of postmenopausal osteoporosis: a review." AM J MED, (1988), 85: 847-850 and D.R. Felson, Y. Zhang, M.T. Hannan, et al., "The effect of postmenopausal estrogen therapy on bone density in elderly women." THE NEW ENGLAND JOURNAL OF MEDI-CINE. (1993), 329: 1141-1146.

2 Darrell W. Brann, "Progesterone: The Forgotten Hormone?" PERSPECTIVES IN BIOLOGY AND MEDICINE. Summer, (1993), 34:4, 642. See also A.I. Csapo and B.A. Resch, "Induction of preterm labor in the rat by the antiprogesterone." AMERICAN JOURNAL OF OBSTETRICS AND GYNE-COLOGY. (1979), 134:823-27.

3 Penelope Ody, THE COMPLETE MEDICINAL HERBAL. (Dorling Kindersley, New York: 1993), 52.

4 Daniel B. Mowrey, THE SCIENTIFIC VALIDATION OF HERBAL MEDICINE. (Keats Publishing, New Canaan, Connecticut: 1986), 112.

5 Lee, 16.

6 Ibid., 52.

7 C. Norman Shealy, M.D., DHEA THE YOUTH AND HEALTH HORMONE. (Keats Publishing, New Canaan, Connecticut: 1996), 34.

8 Lee, 4.

9 Ibid., 101.

10 Ibid., 50.

11 Ibid., 51.

12 Ibid., 101.

13 Ibid., 52.

14 Ibid., See also "Progesterone: Safe Antidote for PMS." MCCALL'S MAGAZINE. October, (1990), 152-56 and Linda Carol Graham, "Do You Have a Hormone Shortage?" REDBOOK. February, (1989), 16.

15 Ibid.

16 Rita Elkins, M.A., DEPRESSION AND NATURAL MEDICINE. (Woodland Publishing, Pleasant Grove, Utah: 1995), 129.

17 Lee, 84.

18 Ibid., 87.

19 Ibid.

20 Alan R. Gaby, M.D., PREVENTING AND REVERSING OSTEOPOROSIS. (Prima Publishing, Rocklin, California: 1994), 150. See also John, R. Lee, M.D. "Osteoporosis reversal: the role of proges-terone." INT CLIN NUTR REV. (1990) 10:3, 384-91 and John R. Lee, M.D., "Osteoporosis reversal with transdermal progesterone." LANCET. (1991), 336, 1327 and John R. Lee, M.D., "Is natural prog-esterone the missing link in osteoporosis prevention and treatment?" MED HYPOTHESES. 35, 316-18.

21 Lee, NATURAL PROGESTERONE, 4.

22 Ibid., 102.

23 Ibid.

24 Shealy, 34.

25 Lee, NATURAL PROGESTERONE, 71. See also R.A.Hiatt, R. Bawol, G.D. Friedman and R. Hoover, "Exogenous estrogen and breast cancer after bilateral oophorectomy." CANCER. (1984), 54, 139-44.

26 Lee, 4. See alsoR.B. Gambrell, "The Menopause: Benefits and Risks of Estrogen-Progesterone Replacement Therapy," FERTIL STERIL, 1983, (37, 457-74).

27 Ibid., 75

28 Ibid., 72. See also, L.D. Cowan, L.Gordis, J. A. Tonascia, and G.S. Jones. "Breast Cancer Incidence in Women with a History of Progesterone Deficiency. JOURNAL OF EPIDIMIOLOGY, 1981, (114) 209.17.

29 Schealy, 35.

30 Ibid..

31 Lee, 74.

32 Schealy, 35.

33 Lee, 102.